In Pursuit of Healing

NAVIGATING THE JOURNEY OF CHRONIC DISEASE

BY DIANA CARUBBA M.D.

SHABAR PUBLICATIONS
www.shabarpublications.com

Published by Shabar Publications
3833 N. Taylor Rd.
Palmhurst, Texas 78573

In Pursuit of Healing! *Navigating the Journey of Chronic Disease*
by Diana Carubba M.D.

Copyright@2024 by Diana Carubba
All rights reserved.
ISBN 978-1-955433-23-5

Most Shabar Publications products *(www.shabarpublications.com)* are available at special quantity discounts for bulk purchase for sales promotions, fund-raising and educational needs.

For details, write Shabar Publications at mayorga1126@gmail.com.

CONTENTS

DEDICATION

I dedicate this book to every patient with the challenge of having a chronic disease.

You are true heroes and brave warriors. You inspire those around you. Because of you, science advances, healthcare teams are developed, and the world moves forward.

The burden you carry is not in vain; hang in there! There is hope for you! Let us navigate this journey together!

ACKNOWLEDGMENTS

To God: He has made me in His image and given me a purpose. I am grateful for life, mercy, and grace, which come only from Him. This book is a gift from Him to all who read it.

To my husband, children, and grandchild: I thrive in the comfort and love of my family and keep going no matter what challenges I face. Because of you, I decided to be strong and courageous and write this book.

To my church family, Hosanna World Changers Church: You are all the ones who stand by me and keep faith and hope alive in me. Thank you for reminding me every day that all we do is part of a more excellent plan designed by God, the creator of the Universe.

To my colleagues in medicine: Only you know what it is to see sickness daily and not get discouraged when treatments fail or patients die. Thank you for helping me carry the burden of chronic disease in our midst.

To David Mayorga: Thank you for believing that through my life and battles, I could deliver a message of hope for all who are yet to be healed. Thank you for the time editing and publishing this book and designing the cover. Without you, this work would not have been possible.

ABOUT THIS BOOK

This book is for patients and healthcare providers who want to explore the maze of chronic disease in greater depth.

It will give understanding and guidance when suffering or taking care of those with a burden of disease that seems to have no end. It will also provide control and autonomy to replace a victim mentality.

I have included and quoted other authors who are experts in different areas of disease management. I recommend that those who desire to delve deeper consult those writings.

I have also presented statistics and scientific studies on areas like sleep hygiene, diets, and lifestyles that have proven to be aids and essential blocks in managing chronic illness.

There is also a section where spirituality is mentioned as an essential part of the healing process. It is not about leading people into a particular religion but about discovering that we are spirit beings in bodies with souls and that every part of us needs healing.

This book also provides tools in the mind/thoughts area,

teaching how important the way we think and what we believe we can or cannot do are. It also teaches how to eliminate specific thinking methods that only delay or arrest the healing process.

Finally, this book will give the patient and healthcare provider the tools needed to move forward every step of the way. It will aid in making comfortable decisions that will create a roadmap to their particular way of healing, allowing them to carry the burden of their disease as best as possible.

You will also find my own experience reflected in these pages as I carry the burden of chronic disease. Testimonials of healing are also included that will bring hope to those who have lost it.

I recommend journaling as you read. Mediating and self-reflecting after every chapter is also helpful for getting the most out of this book.

Share this hope with someone else after reading and celebrating a renewed hope. Let us not be defeated by disease, but let us overcome it.

I hope these notes will accomplish this and much more in you.

FOREWORD

Few understand the challenges of chronic disease better than the author. I met her several years ago when we were both starting our residency training in South Texas, specializing in Internal Medicine. From the beginning, her determination revealed the person she was and the realization that this was just the beginning, even when she had achieved a goal she worked hard to accomplish—starting and then completing her Internal Medicine residency training in the United States of America (USA). She had already achieved a specialty in her home country but was now pursuing Internal Medicine.

I quickly noticed her willingness to help others, even when facing her unique personal and professional challenges, both in life and medicine. She genuinely cared about us, her peers, and her friends, and over the years, I saw her grow into a dedicated physician in a region still in need of profession-als like her. She volunteered to join me in writing and pre-senting a session on teamwork and communication for our first class of medical students at the first medical school based in the Rio Grande Valley. She passionately shared her perspective with these pioneer future physicians, training them to engage with our community, comfort those who suffer, and understand that cure is not always an option.

Her journey is not just one of professional achievement. As she reveals through the pages of her book, she has faced the tribulations of chronic illness within her own family and life. She has lived as a physician, a family member, and an individual and has been there in those battles that come with the practice of medicine and her personal experiences with chronic illness. This book is, in my view, a reflection of her true self—a genuine, caring person dedicated to helping others while finding her paths to healing.

One personal experience stands out to me. I remember how she was there for me as a young physician trying to overcome cultural shock and a relationship breakup as an Internal Medicine resident. This triggered a feeling of isolation and challenged my sense of purpose, but she helped me as she had helped other residents in our program and countless patients.

Whether you share her religious beliefs or have a different sense of spirituality, her stories and reflections will offer wisdom and hope. At the same time, you walk with or directly face your version of chronic illness, whether it's you or someone you love who is suffering or experiencing chronic illness. Her insights on how our thoughts and mindset can help us make better decisions about health and disease reveal her holistic approach to healing.

Her book calls us to understand and define our paths and to make decisions that align with our values and beliefs. Through her experiences, she shares the profound impact of resilience and the human spirit on overcoming adversity.

In Pursuit of Healing: Navigating the Journey of Chronic Disease is for both the religious and the spiritual, as well as anyone seeking to overcome the complexities of chronic illness and find a path through it. It is part of what I think is a life well-lived, filled with compassion, determination, and an unwavering commitment to helping others.

Here are some excerpts from the book to give you a glimpse into the wisdom and insights you will find within these pages. Let her journey inspire you, as it has inspired me:

"I am still trying to figure out if a doctor chooses medicine or medicine chooses a doctor. The doctor's life, my life, soon didn't belong to me anymore. My responsibility as a doctor became what superseded any other call. Even as a wife and a mother, there were instances where I had to leave the comfortable to go into the uncomfortable for others."

"It's like the well-known story of the adult traveling with a child or elderly in an airplane. If the cabin depressurizes, the oxygen masks will immediately be within our reach. The instructions from the airline staff are to put on our oxygen first, then help the help-

less one. We must do that with our bodies if we want to keep carrying loads of life and others. Taking our oxygen first means we must pay attention to the warning signs of our bodies, minds, and emotions to see if things are going in the wrong direction."

"I believe it is the same way with disease. Evidence of disease with signs and symptoms can become so tangled that it is painful, even in the hands of experts in the medical community. Only those that carry diseases that are relentlessly fighting to conquer their bodies and their families know what it is like to see knots everywhere and to wait patiently for those knots to be untangled by someone else."

"Particularly, our emotions are very keen ways to 'know' what's happening inside and outside us. We do need to pay attention to their voice. If we feel sad or discouraged most of the time, there might be an imbalance in our brain neurotransmitters that need adjustments, either with diet, supplements, or medications."

"As you read this last chapter, I want you to consider what you want. Not what your doctor wants, what your daughter wants, or what your spouse wants. It would be best if you decided for yourself. You must take this journey at a time and one day at a time and decide if you want to continue it."

- Jose Campo Maldonado, MD, MSCI, FACP,
Associate Professor UTRGV School of Medicine,
Director of Antibiotice Stewardship VBMC.

INTRODUCTION: *Called to Heal*

My passion for medicine started during middle school. We were neighbors with a medical student who became my older sister's close friend.

After school, he would visit and lay his books on our dining table. He would then talk to us about what it was like to be in medical school. I remember listening, fascinated by his conversations.

But what I loved the most was that after a little while, he would get distracted and talk about other things with my sister and friends. He would then leave his books unattended on the table. This was my great opportunity to discover the treasures kept in those books. The pictures, of course, caught my attention first. Looking at the anatomy of our bodies, I began to yearn to know more about it.

By the time I was in high school, I had made my career choice. In my household, there was no question about whether we would pursue a degree. My mother had made it clear to me and my sisters since elementary school that we would graduate and have a career. So naturally, as soon as high school came, I knew where my path was going.

I got into medical school and graduated with honors. The year before graduation, I completed what was called the Pre-graduate Internship. This was to be a year of hospital experience during which the medical students could practice medicine under the supervision of both residents and mentoring physicians. This began a series of opportunities and experiences that made me a doctor.

In becoming a doctor, I learned about diseases up close. I saw how diseased tissue caused diseased bodies and how, without intervention, death can steal life. I also learned to value life from the womb and to recognize the beauty of a newborn first cry. The tension and excitement of a woman in labor, the suffering with them until their reward arrived, made me not only a spectator but a participant in my patient's lives.

Many stories, maybe thousands of them, compile my now 35 years of practicing medicine. From the beginning years, when I had a safety net of supervising residents and physicians, to the more challenging years of establishing a practice, working for hospitals, and ultimately changing scenery and patient populations, I can now say medicine is still my passion.

I am still trying to figure out if a doctor chooses medicine or medicine chooses a doctor. The doctor's life, my life, soon didn't belong to me anymore. My responsibility as a doctor became what superseded any other call. Even as a wife and a mother, there were instances where I had to leave the comfortable to go into the uncomfortable for others.

But I had made a choice years back, and I was now on a journey that seemed to have no return. I had been called, but now I was also on call. This call had nothing to do with my office schedule or the hospital shift. It had to do with the awareness that there was an enemy, and I was the one to defeat it. Sickness and disease became that enemy. My priority became the healing of others.

Little did I know then that there would be a time in my life when the ancient proverb Physician heal thyself would become true.

I now battle the same enemy, but the battle is not only for others. The enemy got even closer and more defiant than ever as it came to steal health from my own body. Physician heal thyself made me realize that I cannot offer victory to others unless I win this battle for myself.

The journey has started and will only end once there is a winner.

CHAPTER 1

Knowing Your Enemy!: *Defining Disease*

In the race of life, there is always opposition. No matter what background you look at life from, we can all agree that you will encounter barriers or difficulties as you live.

I want to call some of those barriers enemies. Whether physical, mental, or emotional, they all have one purpose: to stop us or at least slow us down in our race in life.

So, if someone or something is not helping me advance, I call that an enemy.

In pursuing healing as a physician, I had to define that enemy. The enemy wasn't the medical bills, the patient's personality, or even the overhead expenses of a practice. The enemy had to be defined; I had to know it fully to defeat it.

So, let us start by knowing our enemy. I am not pretending to present a complete description of every sickness and disease out there. We have excellent resources to learn from every disease's microbiology, pathology, and treatment. I want to define the enemy in another way, a more straightforward but also more comprehensive way.

What is a disease?

Merriam-Webster dictionary defines disease as a condition of the living animal or plant body or of one of its parts that impairs normal functioning and is typically manifested by distinguishing signs and symptoms.

Sickness is defined as ill health (illness), a disorder, a weakened or unsound condition, or a specific disease.

The medical definition by the same dictionary says: an impairment of the normal state of the living animal or plant body or one of its parts that interrupts or modifies the performance of the vital functions, is typically manifested by distinguishing signs and symptoms, and is a response to environmental factors (as malnutrition, industrial hazards, or climate), to specific infective agents (as worms, bacteria, or viruses), to inherent defects of the organism (as genetic anomalies), or to combinations of these factors: sickness, illness, also called Morbus.

It comes from the Middle English disese, from Anglo-French desease, desaise, from des- dis- + eise ease.

I like to think about disease as anything that removes (dis) our ease.

You Know It Is Coming!

Despite all these definitions, our bodies are made so wonderfully that we know when the disease is coming. We are such unique works of art, or you can say technology, science, or whatever pleases you the most, that we have great monitoring systems and alerts when something is going wrong.

But in this world of FAST, fast food, drive-throughs, instant meals, microwaves, etc., it has become difficult to recognize when our bodies are getting sick.

For most of us, life is about being aware of everything around us; we live in an almost paranoid state, thinking about what can go wrong next with everything outside of us.

We are so preoccupied with economics, government, careers, family, etc., that we forget to think about our bodies. I know all the above is extremely important, but functioning correctly as a human being to take care of the rest that calls our attention is essential.

It is like the well-known story of an adult traveling with a child or elderly in an airplane. If the cabin has a depressurization, the oxygen masks will immediately be at our reach. The instructions from the airline staff are to put our oxygen first, then help the helpless one.

We must do that with our bodies to carry life and others. Taking our oxygen first means we must pay attention to the warning signs of our bodies, minds, and emotions to see if things are going in the wrong direction.

Awareness then becomes the number one tool in conquering disease. Knowing our enemy means we must be equipped to recognize it when it is getting close to us and do what we must to stop it before it grows bigger and overpowers us.

Now, some diseases will surprise us. Some congenital problems, cancers, accidents, etc., might not give us warning signs. But many others will, and to be ready, we must recognize the normal state of health from the diseased state.

I compare it to counterfeit money. The banks train the staff to recognize real money first and identify counterfeit money when it arrives.

If we can recognize our state of health, we can be sure that we will identify the enemy of disease when it comes to us. That will give us an advantage when it comes to dealing with it.

Getting to know our bodies, slowing down to be aware of any different symptoms, and recognizing our enemy will prepare us for any healing journey we must take. The race of our lives will one day end, but how we run it will determine our success. Remember, we were wonderfully made!

CHAPTER 2

Are You Just a Body with Problems?:
The Soul, Spirit, and Body Connection

So, how can we detangle this tangle? How do we know where the balance is? How do we detect when something is going wrong?

Answering all these questions is very important if we want to be equipped to fight the battle and win over disease.

Detangling!

I want to start by *detangling*.

When I was a little girl, one of my most feared experiences was what would happen after I showered.

In those days, there was no such thing as washing your body only. Every shower included a hair wash. My hair was and still is very fine. I didn't have much, or at least it didn't seem so, but every time I would come out of the shower, my hair was extremely tangled. I knew what would happen next.

As a little girl, I had no skills to detangle myself, so an adult would have to take over the task. My aunt, who helped raise us, had the task, or another caregiver on the scene.

I would wait and even try to hide to avoid the painful experience. But ultimately, the experience would happen. What makes it interesting is that as my aunt or other caregiver was patiently and as slowly as possible detangling my hair, I was put in front of something nice to distract me and waited patiently.

I especially remember Sunday nights because it was the end of our weekend, and school was early the following day. So, to help me sit patiently through the process, my aunt would put me in front of my favorite TV show and let me stay up a little later.

But everything changed when detanglers came to the scene. One of the trendy beauty product lines then launched a solution in a spray you would apply after showering. The tangles would immediately submit and disappear. It was also made specially for children, so my parents agreed I needed it. What a difference that made to my previously traumatic experiences!

I believe it is the same way with disease. Evidence of disease, with signs and symptoms, can become so tangled that it is painful even for experts in the medical community. Only those who carry diseases that are relentlessly fighting to conquer their bodies and their families know what it is like to see knots everywhere and to wait patiently for someone else to untangle those knots.

The good news is that we don't have to suffer and be simple spectators in detangling. We can participate and use some detangling liquid until we have a clearer idea of what's happening. Again, step number one in conquering and winning is the awareness of ourselves.

I suggest that you think for a minute outside of your preconceived ideas of yourself.

I will present a concept that is not new and is not mine. The idea is that we are not just a body that has problems. We are a three-in-one being. Again, I don't pretend to write about this as an expert, as many other resources go deeper into these truths.

I do want to explain them as simply as possible, though. Then, feel free to dig deeper into them until you accept or reject them. If you take this as truth, it will be like that detangle solution that will help you see clearly and have less pain when dealing with diseases.

I believe in the concept that we are spirits with souls living in bodies.

Our bodies reflect and result from what is happening in the other two realms.

There is an interdependence and interconnection between these three realms of our being.

What happens in one will determine how the other one reacts. The three of them need to be healed to have wholesome health.

Let's look at them separately first; then, we'll integrate them.

The Spirit

Our spirits connect us to God. They are eternal; they will exist forever, and our choices now will determine how our spiritual lives are now and forever.

A strong, healthy spirit will be paramount in our healing journeys.

In quoting King Solomon, he said in the Book of Proverbs: **"The spirit of a man sustains him in sickness, but as for a broken spirit, who can bear it"** (Proverbs 18.14)

So even when disease and sickness assault us, which is inevitable as we live in this world, our spirits can sustain us. We don't want a broken spirit; many circumstances can break spirits.

Spirits can be dormant or weakened by a lack of knowledge and understanding of our spiritual lives. But spirits can also be awakened and enlightened to the understanding of God and the reality of knowing we are spiritual beings.

As we become alive and strong in our spirits, we can receive supernatural strength, wisdom, and counsel when facing opposition to our health.

When we live by the spirit, meaning governed by it, we will not do whatever we desire in our bodies or souls. Someone ruled by the spirit will not give in to things that will damage our bodies or souls. Life in the spirit is excellent and should be developed for us to be stronger and healthier.

I will explain more about keeping our spirits strong in the chapter on prayer. For now, we must consider that neglecting our spiritual needs will eventually make us more vulnerable to diseases.

The Soul

How do we explain the soul realm of our beings? Teachers say it is what we think, feel, and want. Have you ever heard yourself say repeatedly: I think, I want? If you are like most of us, I'm sure you've said it or at least thought it many hundreds or thousands of times. These questions or statements come from the soul part of our beings.

The thoughts, the emotions, and the will are all part of the soul.

This is where it gets complicated. Many of us are wholly driven by the soul. We do what we want, what we think, or what we feel like doing. There's no better recipe for disaster regarding health and healing than letting the soul take control of our lives.

I know your thoughts because I have thought about it multiple times. I have thought thoughts like, "I can trust my gut feeling," "I think this is the solution because I am a thinker and can reason my healing out," or "Today, I feel I can get away with eating what damages me." Yes, it is hazardous to let the soul guide our healing journey. But let's also be fair and not demonize the soul realm.

The soul acts as a gauge of our reality.

Our emotions are keen ways to "know" what's happening inside and outside us. We do need to pay attention to their voices. If we feel sad or discouraged most of the time, there might be an imbalance in our brain neurotransmitters that needs adjustments, either with diet, supplements, or medications.

If we're on edge, nervous, or worried, our bodies might lack hormones or need to avoid certain foods, additives, etc., from our diets. So yes and no. We say yes to our feelings when it comes to acknowledging our symptoms, but we say no to them when they try to distract us from our healing by promoting unhealthy habits.

What about our thoughts? We are marvelous thinking beings. We never stop thinking. There are multiple wonderful resources on the power of our thought life and how to use our minds to heal our bodies.

Our thoughts can become dangerous without the watchful eye of the other two realms, body and spirit.

Our thoughts can become obsessive, and that's a reflection of disease. We can become so focused on specific thoughts that everything else vanishes and lacks importance. Our thoughts can talk to us like a big brother who encourages us or a condemning authority figure. It is essential, then, that the thoughts have a filter where they can be processed. Comparing what we think to wholesome thinking is a must. We cannot rely on our thoughts to always be right. But our thoughts can be recreated as well.

Neuroscientist Caroline Leaf is one of the leading experts on the thought life. Her extensive work and research have made it possible for many people plagued with mental illnesses to stop their medications as they renew their thoughts through her techniques and principles. She states that our thoughts are like trees with many branches. If we have always thought of wrong thoughts, our lives manifest their result. But if, like a good gardener, we recognize the patterns (she calls them strongholds) or our thoughts, we can change them by replacing them with good, positive thoughts that will, in turn, change our lives.

Her work is remarkable. Applying what she's learned can bring healing to our thoughts, which is worth the try.

I could go on and on about this area of thought. For now, it's enough to say go ahead and think. There's nothing worse than a wasteful mind. But think about what you're thinking about. Awareness of our thoughts is the first step to discovering if they're unhealthy and creating chaos. That's the pivotal point where we can accept them as wrong and decide to change.

When it comes to the will part of the soul, it gets even more complicated. This is the part of our soul that protests inside of us and communicates its desires. Ok, so you want to become an entrepreneur. And, of course, that's not bad. But what if you lack the training or knowledge, or, even worse, you're not talented in this arena? The will can become dangerous when it is not filtered against anything else. Returning to our quote from King Solomon, he states in Proverbs that there is safety in the multitude of counselors.

But the will is also crucial to moving us in the right direction, especially regarding healing. We need our will to say yes to that new diet, yes to following our doctor's instructions, yes to stopping our out-of-control activity, and finally, yes to rest.

So, our wills are powerful, like our emotions and thoughts. We cannot separate them since they are all part of our souls. And we cannot ignore them, as our soul is part of who we are.

Author and speaker Joyce Meyer said: "Your emotions (you may include thoughts and will) are just like children. You don't let them drive the car, but you don't put them in the trunk either."

So, let us recognize the importance of our soul in healing our bodies. Unless we pay attention to what's going on within our soul realm, unless we don't ignore it and push it down like it is of no importance, we will have to take a longer road than needed to our healing.

The Body

What can I say about the body component of our beings? There is a reason why I became a doctor: my fascination with the functioning of the human body. We are indeed a marvelous creation.

From the first anatomy lessons to the microbiology, pathology, and physiology lessons, I developed an even greater curiosity to know more about our bodies.

Now, if you remember, at the beginning of the chapter, I said I believe we are spirits, have souls, and live in bodies.

So, our bodies are the shell, if you want to consider it like that. What other people see is what we know about ourselves. The other two realms are more like invisible forces acting from within us and usually manifesting in the reality of our bodies. So, if we are what we and others can see, this is the most potent force that can direct us to pursue and keep pursuing our healing.

When a body is wholesome and healthy, there is a better appreciation of the other two realms. If we are physically healthy, our minds function excellently (most of the time), our thought life tends to be optimistic, and our emotions are well-being. We pursue those things we are most qualified to do, etc.

But if our bodies are sick, our souls and spirits also take a hit.

Being chronically fatigued as part of carrying a chronic illness diagnosis will impair your ability to see yourself as someone productive. It will mess up your thoughts to believe that it is for you. Your will part will be inactive or dormant since you can never seem to complete the tasks ahead of you. Your sick body will also reflect how you think about yourself and others. You will start comparing your body's weight, strength, and abilities to others, worsening things.

So it is of extreme importance, once again, that we become aware of our bodies. In my daily practice of medicine, I treat many patients with diabetes. One of the dreadful complications of this group of patients is something called neuropathy. People with peripheral neuropathy lose the ability to feel, mostly in their feet. They cannot feel pain, vibration, or touch. The worse the diabetes, the worse this symptom is. If you think this is not a big deal, think again. If you suffer from it, I don't have to explain more, but if you don't, let me give you an example of how this symptom can become extremely dangerous.

As these patients are unaware of what happens to their feet, they could step on a rusty nail, cut themselves, and not know it until it is a little too late. By them not feeling the poking of the nail, they can develop an infection of the skin, the bones, and even gangrene that can ultimately require amputation of that foot or leg.

So why do I give this graphic example? Because the same thing can happen to all of us when we are not paying attention to our physical symptoms. Our bodies are created so perfectly that they have integrated alarm systems. We have, for example, fever. Fever tells us there is more than likely an infection going on. Cough tells us something needs to be expelled from our bodies. Fatigue not relieved by regular rest might tell us of an underlying chronic inflammation. We must pay attention to what our bodies are saying. Not doing so will put us on the edge of terrible complications, just like the diabetic with peripheral neuropathy who ignores the nail because he has lost his sensation.

Let us be conscious of what we have in front of the mirror. Aging is standard; some fatigue is normal, especially if we have lost some stamina due to a lack of training in our bodies. But think now and consider: how is my health today compared to last year, the previous month, and last week? Don't just think, "Oh, it is probably that I didn't sleep well," or "It was that pizza that did it." Yes, it might be all the above, but registering a mental or actual diary on paper (or electronic) of your symptoms might be the best gift you can give yourself and your healthcare provider.

A sick body cannot function to its most tremendous potential. Let's be vigilant of all our alarms and do not ignore or neglect them. Healing is ours if we are proactive and conscious of ourselves.

CHAPTER 3

We Are What We Eat . . . For Real!

Do you remember being a kid and eating all sorts of junk food? Yes, those hot summer afternoons spent eating ice cream, snow cones, chips, popcorn, candy, etc.

Do you remember then at night not being hungry for dinner but having stomach pains and maybe even nightmares after eating a whole pizza?

It has been scientifically proven that the kind of food we eat dictates how well our body functions.

It is not my intention in this book to give lectures on nutrition. There are many excellent resources for that. However, I want to emphasize that our amazing bodies need excellent fuel. I can also tell you about my experience trying different "diets" and "protocols."

I recall being in my 30s and working very long hours, then coming home as a single parent to take care of the rest of my responsibilities.

My diet could have been better as I usually eat on the run. I probably only ate breakfast if I could grab a quick breakfast taco from what my dad cooked for my kids or at the gas station. My lunch would consist of any fast food I could find on my way to my job location. Then, for an afternoon "pick me up" snack, I would get a Diet Coke and a chocolate bar. That, for sure, would bring me enough energy to finish the day. Getting home late at night, all I wanted to do was go to bed, but I still had things to do, so my dinner would consist of whatever was left over from my kid's dinner or grab cereal and a banana or perhaps orange juice and a sandwich. Vegetables? Whole grains? Protein? No, none of that for me. But wait, Fridays were special. I would treat the kids to a pizza on Friday night and get some fried wings. That was a treat!

Do any of these scenarios sound familiar to you? The results of my eating habits were noticeable: anxiety, restlessness, racing thoughts, insomnia, fatigue, mind fog...you name it, I had it. But age helped since I could bounce back quickly with naps and an exercise routine at least 4 to 5 times a week. Yes, age and exercise, paired with some rest, worked enough to get me going without getting sick that much.

But turning 40 and then 50 changed all of these. Trying to keep the same pace with the same fuel became extremely difficult. Still, in my 40s, I could accomplish a few things, but I started with symptoms in my body that did not make sense: aching joints, worsening fatigue, depression, less stamina, and less capacity to exercise. Then, in my 50s, it happened! Now, the results of my bad eating habits were manifested.

It was around my 50th birthday when the achy joints now became swollen. I had difficulty completing my days without pain. I had to take extra breaks while seeing patients in my medical practice. I had almost no time to exercise and no desire or strength to do it.

At the start of the day, I had only one thought: when could I return home and rest?

My eating habits mainly stayed the same, except now I ate out of restaurants instead of fast food. My consumption of carbohydrates was large, and vegetables and fruits were rare in my diet.

I kept consuming diet drinks and little water. Then, it became unbearable for my body. I developed a large ovarian tumor that had me in constant pain. Of course, I ignored it most of the time since all my focus was on my medical practice and how to see more and more patients in less time. Accumulation of stress combined with an inferior diet gave me a 10x10 cm ovarian tumor.

I remember a couple of times during my practice hours feeling so exhausted that I had to be taken to the ER department across the street, only to be discharged with an "Extreme Exhaustion" diagnosis. Did that change my habits? NO!

Once the ovarian tumor was diagnosed in one of those ER trips, I started to recognize that something I was doing was not right faintly. Maybe I could change my situation if I could make some changes. I ended up needing almost emergency surgery to remove that giant mass in my pelvis.

The gynecologist on call realized that the mass could be cancer and referred me to a gynecologist-oncologist as an emergency. The ovary was removed, and it was benign, but in my surgeon's opinion, it was already behaving like cancer, and he had a hard time removing it from the other organs. The recovery was hard and long, but I returned to my practice without making any changes.

Of course, the damage to my body had begun many years prior, and it continued as I did not make any changes to my diet/exercise/stress levels.

Now, my joints were killing me. Stiffness, swelling, fatigue, pain, all these symptoms progressed to the point of making me miss workdays. Only then did I start to look for solutions. I went to a few doctors until finally, one of them diagnosed me with Rheumatoid Arthritis.

I began different medications, many with terrible side effects. My doctor patiently started going through his armament of drugs to see which was the one that would be effective enough to control my symptoms but gentle enough not to cause me unbearable side effects.

In the middle of all this, I came across one book that a patient recommended. She had Multiple Sclerosis and was being treated by a neurologist in the community. She said to me that when she started eating differently, her symptoms dramatically improved and that even her neurologist was amazed at the changes and the less need for medications. I was desperate for relief, so I immediately purchased a copy and began the journey to the "Wahls Protocol."

This protocol diet was developed by a physician diagnosed with Multiple Sclerosis. She discovered that many foods we consume are pro-inflammatory, but many are anti-inflammatory. With that in mind, she developed a system in which, depending on your level of inflammation or disease, you escalate a system or protocol to increase the anti-inflammatory foods and decrease the pro-inflammatory ones. In a nutshell, I had to leave the foods I loved and craved and start eating foods that were foreign to my body and that I did not like.

I forced myself into this new way of eating. It became more frustrating than anything since now I had to cook, I did not eat at restaurants anymore, and I was constantly hungry many times. But I stuck to it for a while, and I started noticing my mind fog disappearing, my joints were not swollen, I had the energy to exercise, and the pain was almost gone.

As a doctor, I, of course, attributed the improvement to a better medication regimen. So slowly but surely, I began to stray away from my healthy eating habits. Going back to bad is always easy, so I was almost back where I had started.

Reintroducing the old food did give me a wake-up call as I discovered that, indeed, the new food choices had made a difference in some symptoms of my disease.

Since then, I have tried different things. I knew that "protocol" had helped me, but I wasn't willing to give up some food pleasures even when the results were modest to good.

Multiple scientific studies prove that such and such food is terrible and such and such food is good. Many prove remarkable results, but then we must consider which population they used, whether this applies to my circumstances, whether I am the right age or have the right disease, whether I exercise like them, etc.

Your body is a remarkable creation that does extraordinary things and should be treated respectfully.

We should ingest those foods that we respond best to. Suppose any bread, whether sprouted or organic, bloats me if it is wheat, then no wheat. If I have a problem with berries, even when proven to give us great brain benefits, I should not eat them.

Sticking to a diet, a formula, or a protocol is only sometimes the best idea. I am not saying you should not try it; by all means, I am all for trying new things, but we should always design those according to our body's response.

If we are doing great without dairy, stay without it for a while. Most experts recommend at least 6 - 12 months of stopping an offending food before introducing it again and seeing if those sensitivities have disappeared. It is different with food allergies. Those should not be consumed again unless you are under the supervision of an Allergy specialist and are desensitized through vaccines or any other modality.

Eating is not just for survival; it is also considered a pleasure and a social activity. We should try our best to give our bodies the proper fuel for food and make it pleasurable and socially inviting.

CHAPTER 4

Breaking-Up is Hard to Do!:
Breaking Old Habits, Forming New Habits

In the previous chapter, we discussed how food impacts health. This is nothing new. The concept of eating healthy and its consequences are well known by almost anyone we can talk to.

Everyone has tried this or that diet or has been a vegan, pescatarian, or keto enthusiast.

But what about other things that can benefit or destroy our health?

Food is only one of many factors that contribute to us being sick or healthy.

I want us to cover other things that can also hinder our healing journey, including habits.

The title of this chapter almost sounds like a country song, and country songs are known for being sad most of the time. As we discuss habits and how they influence us, we will recognize that one of the hardest things to do is break a habit.

Everyone will be very familiar with the concept of addiction and how it goes beyond a habit and becomes an entangling situation that prevents us from becoming our best versions of ourselves.

But if we take a notch lower, we can see that other activities, ways of thinking, and preferences in our daily lives can also entangle and prevent us from achieving our desired goals of healing and healthier living.

For teaching purposes and to categorize them, we will call these habits.

Let's talk about a few of them.

1. The habit of wrong thinking.
2. The habit of indecision.
3. The habit of people-pleasing.
4. The habit of insecurity.
5. The habit of saving others.
6. The habit of over-working.
7. The habit of unforgiveness.

All of these have one thing in common: the difficulty in first recognizing it as a habit damaging us and, second, exchanging it for new habits.

Bad Habits We Must Recognize!

1. *The Habit of Wrong Thinking.*

In the Bible, a Proverb states, "As a man thinks in his heart, so is he." Our behaviors result from the way we think. We act on our thoughts, and often, we don't even take the time to think; we act on our impulses.

Training our minds to think is extremely important for healing. Many techniques and practices now consider our thinking patterns a way of healing our minds, emotions, and bodies.

Thinking the right thing at the right time can make a significant difference in us. It all starts with our perceptions of who we are and our thoughts. If we think of ourselves as someone who will always be sick or who has this or that disability, then we will reflect that in our bodies.

I am not talking about denying reality and healing ourselves by constantly thinking about it. How we approach our current situation with our thoughts can make a difference.

Dr. Caroline Leaf exposes the science of thoughts in her best-selling book Who Switched Off My Brain. She states that our behaviors come from our thoughts, and our thoughts come from our experiences. She describes how thought is formed and stays with us, creating a tree made of branches or experiences. She also states that our thoughts can be changed by changing how we perceive our experiences and creating new thoughts that replace old or damaging ones. Based on this premise, she now has helped many who suffer from mental health issues, from anxiety to depression to addictions and behavioral problems, without any medications!

It all starts with the way we think. In her New York Times best-selling classic Battlefield of the Mind: Winning the Battle in Your Mind, speaker and author Joyce Meyer describes how our thoughts are critical to our behavior and relationships. She describes ways of thinking that can trap us in a state of mind not conducive to our personal best. She also gives tools to overcome those patterns to see the results we want and improve our lives.

In a nutshell, thinking the right thoughts produces the right results. If we want to see healing in our lives, we must break the habit of wrong thinking and start the habit of correct thinking.

2. *The Habit of Indecision.*

Are you a procrastinator? There is nothing worse than staying in a place where no decisions are made. Decisions must be made whenever we want to move forward in our lives.

There are people known as risk takers, cautionary, and safe. But even if you fall into either of those categories, we all experience times of indecision.

The problem with indecision is when it becomes a habit. Indecision is not good; it prevents us from accomplishing those things that benefit us and others.

When we cannot make decisions, we know what we will get: the same thing we already have.

The habit of indecision impacts our healing journey tremendously. I am talking now to those of us who carry the burden of a chronic or incurable disease. Many diseases are now considered incurable by science alone. The hope of healing decreases or is eliminated by simply hearing this prognosis. Right in that place, indecision can creep in uninvited and settle in our minds like an old friend. That is why recognizing and eliminating this trick from its roots is so important.

We always have choices: the choice to pursue healing or not, the choice to see this doctor or that doctor, and the choice to accept or deny this treatment. Traditional medicine wants to eliminate those choices and leave the sick unenabled. But if we can beat this indecision habit by making small choices, we can become empowered and regain hope.

Indecision occurs when we are afraid of the unknown in our healing journey. Indecision habits can be overcome by getting informed. Awareness of what science, traditional medicine, and nontraditional medicine have to say about our diagnosis will give us the strength to make decisions.

Whether this decision leads to victories or not, staying active and advancing in our journeys is essential.

3. The Habit of People Pleasing

Nothing is worse than doing things to please others at the cost of not doing what we must to get well. Of course, we all like to please others, which is good to some extent. We all want to be liked, accepted, and appreciated; sometimes, the way to get those things is to go above and beyond to please those around us.

Many people with chronic and especially autoimmune diseases are considered people pleasers.

Dr. Gabor Mate, in his book The Myth of Normal, describes that in different scientific studies, it was shown that people who suffer from autoimmune diseases are the most admirable patients, those who don't complain, and are overall the most excellent patients, as per the doctor and his staff. These patients are generally people pleasers. They will not stand up for themselves or contradict their doctor's opinions just to be liked by them and feel accepted. This is a very high price to pay for our healing. Whether this behavior precipitates the autoimmune disease or contributes to it must be dealt with if it means victory over it.

So, next time we are tempted to comply with our diagnosis, treatment, prognosis, or any other doctor or health practitioner's recommendations, we must ask ourselves if this is what we want.

Being our best advocate will pay off. It will heal our bodies and souls.

4. The Habit of Insecurity.

Being insecure comes with having a chronic disease. The lives of those living with chronic diseases become centered around the disease. There is a shift in their worlds, and the disease burden is now taking center stage. This can make even the most secure person insecure.

The first step in dealing with insecurity is to conduct a self-inventory and determine whether it is present.

We might feel like we are still in control and, on the outside, pretend and look secure enough. But if we are honest, our insides tell a different story. Feelings of insecurity can come and go, and that is fine. We must let them be there, process them, and then decide that that's not who we are and push them away.

Our security must come not from how well our bodies and minds function but from who we are. This journey can be challenging but enjoyable.

The journey of self-discovery is happening during the disease. To cite again, Dr. Gabor Mate, in *The Myth of Normal*, presents cases of patients even with incurable diseases who discovered themselves in the process of their diseases and even considered the disease as a gift.

As we travel this disease journey, we should take it as an opportunity to discover ourselves and be secure in who we are, not in what we do, as many diseases will impair our job performance. Let us fight this habit of insecurity by thinking every day about how this disease allows us to reevaluate ourselves. Our value is in who we are.

5. *The Habit of Saving Others.*

If you have ever traveled on an airplane, you know the flight attendants' routine instructions. They always go through the safety features in the plane, emergency exits, etc. But they always emphasize that if you are traveling with a child or an elderly person and the cabin gets depressurized, you must put on your oxygen mask first and then take care of the person next to you.

As people who have developed a chronic disease, we carry personality trends. The caregiver personality will look at their surroundings and always find someone to take care of.

Sometimes, this, even when very selfless and generous, can lead the sick person to forget about themselves and keep doing things for others even when their physical or mental stamina is not there.

As we face chronic diseases, whether autoimmune or not, we should consider returning to ourselves and taking care of ourselves first. Taking care of others first might be entrenched in us, and it may become a lifestyle we cannot be without. But it must be broken as a habit and replaced by a healthier one.

Seeing ourselves as superheroes to everyone else may initially be satisfying. Still, it can become a heavy burden and even cause resentment toward those we care for.

However, finding a balance is never too late; we can still love and care for others, but we should begin by loving ourselves. As our love tanks are filled, we can care for and love others out of the overflow. We should remember to take our oxygen first.

6. The Habit of Overworking.

You will have a different working style depending on what generation you were born in. The generations in the workforce include the traditionalists (born between 1925 and 1945), the baby boomers (1946-1964), Gen X (1965-1980), Millennials (1981-2000), and Gen Z (2001-2020).

People who have studied their work styles have seen marked differences, from their loyalty to their tech savvy. But no matter which generation you were born in, there should be a place for rest. People who overwork do not give their bodies and minds a break. It is like keeping a car going on a gas tank and expecting it to keep going and going and going.

Our bodies are not machines or robots; we have cells that are alive, reproduce, and die.

Overworking can stress the cells and their mechanisms to the point of developing or perpetrating disease. Overworking can also turn into workaholism, which is a form of addiction to work with all the behaviors and consequences of a substance or action dependence.

Overworking will prevent our healing and damage our relationships with others and ourselves.

This habit must be recognized to be able to deal with it. Replacing it with a good habit of rest and leisure time might be difficult initially, but it will undoubtedly give us a great reward and promote our healing.

7. The Habit of Unforgiveness

Author and speaker Joyce Meyer has said that unforgiveness is like drinking poison expecting to harm somebody else. This is a perfect picture of what unforgiveness does to our souls. We know now that if our souls are sick, our bodies will be ill.

When someone has hurt us, our reaction is to get offended. Offenses can come in many shapes or forms; some are real, but some are imaginary. We might get offended by someone who did not intend to offend us. It does not matter if this offense is real or not, but what matters is the effect of the offense. It will take root in our souls and become bitter if not dealt with. Bitterness then can cause anger that can be internalized if not expressed healthily.

When bitterness, anger, self-pity, and hatred develop, then many physical and mental symptoms can develop as well.

The proper action when we tend to hold on to unforgiveness

is the opposite: forgiveness!

To forgive someone for the wrong done to us does not make that wrong right, but it does release us from the experience and help us heal. The person or situation that offends does not need to be reconciled to us, and relationships do not have to be restored to give forgiveness.

We must forgive ourselves for past mistakes, recognize how we have hurt others, and ask for forgiveness.

Forgiveness is then like cleaning the slate, erasing the blackboard, deleting the computer data, and starting afresh.

CHAPTER 5

Charge Mode: *The Importance of Sleep*

What happens when you don't get a good night's sleep? Do you remember ever having one? Perhaps you currently struggle with getting enough rest at night. Or have you ever experienced working the "graveyard shift"?

In any of those scenarios, one thing is common to all: not sleeping enough equals less energy the following day to perform the tasks you usually perform.

When I was a medical resident, we spent long hours awake. Not only did we have to be awake, but most importantly, we had to make medical decisions and sometimes perform medical procedures. All of these required very sharp and focused minds.

I did two medical residencies in my career, the first in Mexico and the second in the U.S. In the first one, I was in my late 20s, and the second one was in my mid-40s. However, age was not the only factor in the equation; you might think that I had more strength, stamina, and focus despite being awake for many hours because I was younger in the first one. Still, the truth is that what made the difference was the hours I had to be awake while doing my training.

You see, by the time I did my residency training in the U.S., they had already conducted research after research about the capacity of medical residents to work safely with fewer hours of sleep.

A particular study found in the article "NIOSH Training for Nurses on Shift Work and Long Work Hours" on the Center for Disease Control (CDC) website showed that:

- Being awake for 17 hours is similar to having a blood alcohol concentration of 0.05%.

- Being awake for 24 hours is similar to having a blood alcohol concentration of 0.10%.

This and many other research studies show what anyone who has worked graveyard shifts or has been awake for many hours knows: lack of sleep puts you in a state of deprivation very similar to that of someone who has been intoxicated with a substance.

The opposite is true: the more relaxing and refreshing sleep is, the more we function.

In an article in The Magazine (2018) by Christopher M. Barnes, Sleep Better, Lead Better, it states that in a study by the National Health Interview Survey, the percentage of Americans getting no more than six hours a night rose from 22% in 1985 to 29% in 2012.

An international study conducted in 2017 by the Center for Creative Leadership found that the problem is even worse among leaders: 42% get six or fewer hours of sleep a night. The author conducted studies showing that when a boss or manager did not get restorative sleep of at least 6 hours per night, their performance and relationships with their direct reports were negatively affected.

That's why many corporations, such as Google, Zappos, and Price Waterhouse Coopers, embrace naps during work time to improve employee productivity and efficiency.

More American leaders have now adopted napping, which has traditionally been in place by Japan, with the inemuri or napping at work viewed positively. Spain has also tradition-ally encouraged employees to take naps during the day. Sleep is considered a priority in the workplace today to be a more successful leader.

Other benefits of a good night's sleep are health benefits. In an article published in Healthline by Joe Leech, MS and reviewed by Nick Villalobos, M.D. in 2023, 10 Reasons to Get More Sleep, it was found that:

1. Multiple studies have linked obesity to a lack of restorative sleep of at least 7 hours per night. Sleep deprivation increases appetite and cravings for high-sugar and high-fat foods due to increased levels of gherkin (the hormone that makes us feel hungry) and decreased levels of leptin (the hormone that makes us feel full).

2. It improved concentration and productivity. A study that focused on overworked physicians found that those with moderate, high, and very high sleep-related impairments were 54%,96%, and 97% more likely to report clinically significant medical errors. In children, it can improve academic performance.

3. Maximize athletic performance: Sleep enhances fine motor skills, reaction time, muscular power, endurance, and problem-solving skills.

4. May strengthen your heart: An analysis of 19 studies found that people who slept less than 7 hours had a 13% increased risk of death from heart disease. Another study showed that people who slept less than 5 hours per night had a 61% higher risk of developing high blood pressure than those who slept 7 hours.

5. Sugar metabolism and type 2 Diabetes risk: Sleep deprivation increases insulin resistance. An analysis of 36 studies showed that sleeping less than 5 hours or fewer than 6 hours increased the risk of developing diabetes by 48% and 18%, respectively.

6. Depression: In a study of 2,672 participants, it was found that those with anxiety and depression reported poorer sleep scores than those without anxiety and depression.

7. Healthy Immune System: In one study, participants who slept less than 5 hours were 4.5 times more likely to get a cold than those who slept more than 7 hours. Other studies suggest proper sleep improves the body's antibody response to the influenza vaccine.

8. Inflammation: Sleep loss activates inflammatory signaling pathways, with increased levels of markers of inflammation

like interleukin-6 and C-reactive protein. Chronic inflammation can cause the development of other diseases, such as cancer, Alzheimer's, depression, and type 2 diabetes.

9. Emotional and social interactions: Lack of sleep makes us more prone to emotional outbursts and affects our ability to respond to humor and show empathy. Also, those who are chronically sleep-deprived are more likely to withdraw from social events and experience loneliness.

10. The danger of sleep deprivation: The CDC (Center for Disease Control) reported that 1 in 25 people have fallen asleep while driving. Those who slept fewer than 6 hours were most likely to fall asleep while driving. Another study in 2018 found that the risk of a car accident increases with each hour of lost sleep.

It is then of extreme importance that we consider sleep as part of our healing journey.

As we sleep better, our bodies respond better to pharmacological and non-pharmacological approaches to treating our conditions.

So, next time you cannot sleep or feel tired after sleeping

enough hours, consider what is provoking your lack of rest, discuss it with others who have been there and have successfully overcome this, and get your daily dose of ZZs adjusted.

CHAPTER 6

Different Doctors, Different Mindsets:
The Art of Medicine

There are a myriad of approaches to diagnosing and treating diseases. Yes, most diseases have certain diagnostic tools and specific treatment protocols. But let's face it: medicine is as much science as art.

An artist knows what he will create; it is inside of him. All he must do is select his tools to create the masterpiece. The masterpiece will be unique to him because it came out of him. Even in an art school, different artists will paint or make the same piece of art, and they will look different. I believe in medicine, and something similar happens.

You can have the same disease, but every practitioner will give it their perspective.

This is where medicine turns from science to art. Many will not agree with me and insist that the number of clinical trials and the mathematical equations describing how efficient a drug or treatment is should guide our thinking as physicians. In statistics, it might look like the real thing. But what about that 1% of the population that did not respond? What about those who failed the mathematical equation and decided to be unique?

As unique as a person is, the physician should be unique.

This is not to say that we all do what we think is best, but that we consider all that science and research have done and mix it with our experience, compassion, and uniqueness in treating our patients.

I am grateful that doctors are made in different ways. One patient might need a stern, firm, and controlling doctor, while another might need a more patient, flexible, and compassionate one. Patients might need both styles in their doctors during different seasons or diseases.

My mother had a saying every time she would see her doctor. She might have been feeling very sick, but the moment she saw her doctor come into the room, she would always say, the moment I see you is the moment I get better. This is the best translation I can do from her Spanish.

Now, she did not greet all her doctors like that. My mother had a way of selecting who would be her doctor and who would not. She had to like them, she said. The doctor my mother preferred was the one that 1) had a smile on their face, 2) could listen to her without interruptions, and 3) would agree with her care plan. She also preferred them to be good-looking and would always compliment those good looks.

At the end of her life, her last doctor was an oncologist whose first language was Portuguese, who spoke English with a strong accent. My mother spoke a bit of English and understood most of it, but she could not communicate with him as she liked to. Their relationship could have been better.

My sisters and I had to be in the room to interpret and consistently convey the proposed care plan. But until the end, she remained in control of her medical care. She decided to stop all treatments and chose the hospice route at the end of her life. I can say her doctor had at least 2 out of the three characteristics my mother was looking for in a physician: he did smile, and he finally agreed to stop aggressive medical therapy and accepted the hospice decision. He did not let my mother talk much; my family or I always guided the conversations.

In her article Art of Medicine, Art as Medicine, and Art for Medical Education published in the Canadian Medical Education Journal, author Patricia Lynn Dobkin emphasizes the importance of considering medicine an art, but also how art can be medicine and how future doctors benefit from participating in the arts during their medical education.

She defines the art of medical practice as a clinician's way of being when interacting with patients and families. How doctors, nurses, and allied health care professionals (HCPs) diagnose, explore treatment options, communicate, and promote healing are examples of the art of medicine.

In my own story, being treated by different physicians has made me realize that not everything we see is visible.

A young neurologist in Mexico told me that the eyes will not see what the brain does not know. She was referring to how she was directly approaching my condition and how others might not have seen what she was indeed seeing in me. It has something to do with knowledge but much to do with art.

She also told me of a story when she had just graduated from her neurology residency when the COVID pandemic hit. She said most of the neurologists in the city of Monterrey, Mexico, where she practices, were over 60 years old, and most preferred not to be exposed to the virus, so they stopped attending the hospitals. She, however, continued to take care of patients. She said that at one point, she had to stop looking at her medical books and start thinking for herself about what to do. The newness of this pandemic and how the bodies were responding to the virus made her realize that she would be losing patients' lives unless she practiced medicine as an art.

Suppose you are not a physician but a patient. In that case, you need to be comfortable and secure that those treating you are using not just their head knowledge, not just the statistics and numbers, but that they consider your uniqueness as the defining factor in approaching your condition.

If you are a physician, consider the privilege to take life into your hands and make decisions that can alter their course.

As we incorporate all our beings into the equation, the result will be much more favorable than seeing a diagnosis and prescribing a drug or procedure to fix it.

We as physicians should not be considered as fixers of a disease but more as participants in the elaborate process of bringing wholeness to an individual's reality.

As participants, our vantage point is limited by our knowledge and reasoning but very important for the results.

Let us then consider that if we use medicine as art and art as medicine, we can become those who will promote healing in others and be made whole in the process.

CHAPTER 7

The Great Physician: *The Power of Prayer!*

I have had the great privilege of being a missionary doctor. I remember when my friend's nurse asked me if I wanted to go on a mission trip to Jamaica. Before even thinking about it, my mouth said yes. I had no idea how that yes would transform my life and how I saw medicine forever.

I am a woman of faith, and throughout my medical career, I have made it a point to share that faith with the sick to give them hope beyond medical science.

I therefore believe in prayer changing circumstances and even outcomes. I have been a witness to different manifestations of the power of prayer. I also have multiple examples of what prayer has done for the sick and those involved in their care.

When it comes to healing, all is fair. People who are subjected to diseases, especially chronic or fatal ones, will go above and beyond to regain their health. Often, these patients will gladly receive prayers if offered.

I was not always a doctor who prayed, but that changed when

I was born with my faith in Jesus of Nazareth. As I read the multiple healing stories through prayer, something in me changed. I also wanted to bring that kind of healing to others.

Science is usually predictable, and we know what to expect from treatments, including drugs, physical modalities, surgical interventions, etc. However, the prayer of faith could restore a patient with or without the other interventions. So, more guided by compassion than by faith, I started to regularly include the practice of praying for my patients.

I don't remember if any of them declined prayer when offered, maybe one with a particular faith that almost prohibited a woman from praying. I did not always offer to pray directly, as circumstances were different, but I did when the scenario was appropriate.

As I said, I am not trying to list all the answered prayers or even the miracles I have witnessed right now. I want to mention some of them that impacted me and encouraged me to keep doing what I was doing.

I was in my residency training in Internal Medicine when I saw something I could not believe. As I was rounding on my patients, one of them was going for surgery for a leg amputation. I offered prayer, and he agreed; I thought my prayer would be for safe surgery, a good outcome, etc., but instead, out of my mouth, I commanded new circulation to this leg in the name of Jesus. I did not feel anything strange, nor did my prayer sound powerful. I do know that I was surprised when those words came out of me. I left the patient's room and continued my morning duties. About 2 hours later, all the residents were called to the classroom. This was not a scheduled lecture, but we were told to get there as soon as possible; the interventional cardiologist came and said he had just witnessed something that he could not explain. He said this man was scheduled for an amputation this morning, but before he was taken, he had this study again, and we found his circulation had been restored to normal. Then he added, And there's no natural explanation for what happened. I couldn't believe what I was hearing and did not dare say anything. I knew that prayer had done something supernatural in this man.

Another supernatural healing occurred to someone very close to me.

My younger sister was in labor for the first time after multiple attempts at getting pregnant. She delivered a healthy baby boy, and we were all rejoicing. But things did not develop as expected, and she began to bleed profusely. I was called back to the hospital to help my brother-in-law make a decision that would determine if my sister would live or die. The decision was made to proceed with surgery to remove her uterus. She was in a state called DIC, meaning her blood was not clotting appropriately, and she was bleeding to death. Surgery would suggest trying to save her life by removing her uterus, but she could die from the bleeding anyway during the surgical intervention. The doctor intervening explained that she was already in a comatose state, unconscious due to the blood loss, and she was already in kidney failure as well. Her liver was starting to fail, also. We decided that the best option was to do something, and he took her to surgery.

I asked if I could pray for her. I had called someone else before going to the hospital to help me pray, so I prayed nonstop on my way to the hospital. The doctor agreed, and he and his staff joined me in prayer. My sister looked dead already; she was swollen, her skin was greenish/pale, and she was oozing blood from her IV lines. She was cold as ice. When I said amen, I looked around and saw everyone who had prayed with me. She was taken to the operating room, and I went back to pray by myself.

What happened next is also considered supernatural, but in my faith, I believe God was already answering our prayers; I saw a vision of my sister on the operating table with the doctors and nurses around her, but the image of Jesus hovering on top of her. And I could hear Him say I will save her life, and she will dance for Me. I knew at that moment my sister would be ok.

When the doctor came out, he reassured us the surgery went well, but we would have to wait for the outcome since my sister was already in bad shape before surgery, and only time would tell if she would recover her mind, her kidneys, and her liver.

The following day, I called the hospital, and my aunt answered the phone; she looked after my sister and said, Do you want to talk to her? I was so surprised that she could speak that I rushed from work to the hospital to see her. When I got to the hospital, the doctor was on his way out, and he stopped to show me my sister's new blood results. He said, "I have no explanation for what happened; all her results are normal, and she is awake. It must have been the prayers; no scientific explanation exists."

These are only two examples of what I have seen regarding the power of prayer.

I am not the only one who has experienced this, and I recommend that you read other significant publications on prayer and healing, like Randy Clark's *Power to Heal* and John G. *Lake's Divine Healing*.

Many scientific studies are researching the power of prayer in healing.

In a study published by Chittaranjan Andrade in the Indian Journal of Psychiatry in 2009, *Prayer and Healing: A Medical and Scientific Perspective on Randomized Controlled Trials*, several other studies were analyzed, and some showed positive outcomes for prayer while others did not. Some of these studies were done in animals, eliminating the placebo effect. They concluded that it would be challenging to include all potential variables in every study to compare whether prayer was part of the outcomes. It could be they said the time spent in prayer, the quality of the prayer, and ultimately, the decision of the divine entity addressed to grant the prayer or not.

Ultimately, can divine healing be considered science? A new research field called neurotheology shows that the brains of people who spend time in prayer and meditation are different. The changes that occur in our brains as we pray are called neuroplasticity. Dr. Caroline Leaf has shown that brain changes can be seen on brain scans after practicing prayer and meditation over eight weeks.

But before discussing the power of prayer, we must consider the Biblical premise that the prayer of faith will heal the sick.

As we pray, we must have faith that Someone more significant and powerful than ourselves will hear that prayer and answer according to what He has promised to deliver. That is called faith; we can ask for it if we don't have it.

As I started sharing in this chapter, my life as a doctor who prays and believes in great outcomes was changed as I traveled as a missionary to Jamaica. In countries where healthcare is so limited, a greater level of faith in prayer increases to the point that healing and miracles occur.

As we physicians also encounter limited possibilities in healing through science, our faith in the supernatural can increase to the level of daring faith.

Believing in supernatural outcomes might take a lot of work. Still, as we continue to include them in our arsenal of weapons against disease, we might have different eyes to see other realities.

Let us not discount the possibilities the sick have when achieving complete restoration of their health. Let us consider prayer part of them and start using it more rather than less.

CHAPTER 8

Do You Want to Get Well?: *Making a Decision*

The title of this chapter might sound like a joke. Of course, we want to get well! But let me start by telling a story that goes back to the times of the Bible. I am referring to an encounter Jesus of Nazareth had with a sick person. The question Do you want to get well? has such wisdom that it deserves to be answered by the originator of that question, the great Physician Jesus Christ of Nazareth.

Jesus encounters a man lying by a pool of healing waters for 38 years.

In this pool, an angel stirred the waters at appointed times. Many people lay around, some blind, some lame, some withered, all waiting for the waters to stir. The first one to go in would be healed.

When Jesus sees this man and knows he has been there for a long time, He asks the famous question: Do you want to get well? If Jesus knew all things, then He knew the man was there due to a physical ailment that had him paralyzed for 38 years.

Despite this, His question is directed at the sick man. What happens after is the reason for writing this chapter. The paralytic man starts giving Jesus excuses because he has not been healed so far. His reply goes like this: I have no one to put me in the water, and when I try to get in, someone else gets ahead of me. Jesus' response is simple: get up, pick up your mat, and walk. And the man did.

Rather than preaching a sermon to you, I want us to consider possible similarities between that man and you.

What I am about to describe next might make some uncomfortable. I want to uncover areas we need to be aware of in our healing.

In my healing journey, I have had to discover some of these areas, and most of the time, it was not a pleasant discovery but one that required me to be transparent and honest. It also required me to acknowledge those areas and to make a decision.

In saying this, I am now disclosing that I will be as tender as possible and firm as needed to keep our hope for healing alive.

The paralytic man lying in that pool for 38 years can inspire us to look at ourselves and our healing. His answer tells us a lot about his personality. A personality he developed as he was sick for so many years. I can describe it as:

1. Dependent personality: the paralytic man, due to his inability to fend for himself, had developed a dependent personality. He knew that to get anything, he had to depend on others. He probably had gotten used to it. But maybe he also had become aware that he was a burden to others. He knew he needed others, but throughout the years, many probably had rejected him or had been physically or emotionally unavailable to meet his personal needs. As he lay there, he expected others to help him and found no one. He had a good excuse for not getting into the waters. The solution was right before him, but he did not get it because of a lack of help. As we travel our healing journey, we might feel that no one can help us. Let me tell you that is a lie. There will be people around us that we can count on to make the journey easier. But we must also not depend on others to get to our destinations. We must try to use all available resources and within our reach. We might be paralyzed in some form or another. We might be limited in our bodies or our minds. Our emotions might need most of the restoration. But there is always something we, ourselves, can do about it. It might be a phone call or going outside to meditate or enjoy the peaceful scenery, but we all can do something for ourselves to get to that place of healing.

2. *False identity:* The paralytic man had changed how he looked at himself. For 38 years, he could not move from his mat without the help of others. I believe before he was paralyzed, he had dreams of his future. He probably wanted to marry and have a family. I don't know if he did, but I am sure that throughout the years, his dreams started to die, and finally, he remained by that pool, waiting and waiting. While waiting for our healing, our minds can talk to and tell us different stories about ourselves. If we think of ourselves as someone strong, someone wise, someone with determination, sickness can tell us we are weak and dumb and lack the perseverance to complete our goals and ambitions. Our personality can change so much that we no longer know who we are. We now become "the sick person," we become "the paralytic," and we become "the woman with arthritis, diabetes, multiple sclerosis, or whatever diagnosis you might have. You were that same person before you got diagnosed; you have not lost the ability to dream, plan, and do whatever makes you unique. The moment you start seeing yourself as the sick person, you become the ill person. But that is not who you are; that is just a result of your condition. We need to hang on to who we indeed are. We can do that by remembering and

keeping images of ourselves of times when the disease had not taken over our lives. Dodie Osteen, the mother of Joel Osteen, in her book Healed of Cancer, says that one of the things that kept her going in her journey was to have pictures of herself enjoying life and doing activities that she could not do while battling the disease. That kept her grounded on who she was and not on a false identity of being sick.

3. *Self-pity:* As we look at ourselves with different eyes, we move from being compassionate to having self-pity. That is if we must be more careful and aware of this potentially horrible complication. To have compassion and empathy for ourselves is very important. We can't look at ourselves with negative emotions like anger, unforgiveness, shame, guilt. We might feel guilty or responsible for having the disease. We really must look at ourselves and acknowledge our responsibility. In the case of diseases like diabetes or hypertension, for example, weight plays a significant role, as does the way we eat. So, in that case, looking at what we do and how our decisions play an important role in controlling the disease is essential. But after doing that, there is no benefit in feeling guilty about it. We must recognize our part in it and then decide to change. Guilt must go along with shame for what we did or did not do to contribute to the development of the disease. Then we have compassion for ourselves; we

treat ourselves as if we were treating any other sick person. We recognize our limitations at the time, and we move according to them. I know it is not easy; many emotions will surface, such as frustration, anger, and sadness, to name a few. But if those emotions have an excellent outflow, it is ok for us to manifest them. It is good that we do that. Bottling up our feelings will only guarantee they will explode most inappropriately and cause more damage than good. But what we don't want is to end up having pity for ourselves. If we become so self-absorbed in our misery, we will stay miserable. Looking at everything we have lost instead of on the lessons we are learning will make us sad, depressed, and feel sorry for ourselves. That can consume us to the point of not having any hope for restoration of our health. To recognize self-pity, ask yourself these questions:

- Am I getting comfortable with the idea of being sick all the time?

- Do I like the extra attention I get because I am now ill and dependent on others?

- Have I come to the point where I don't expect healing anymore, so I don't look for opportunities/ ways of getting better?

Any yes to those might be a sign that self-pity is luring around us to get us into the trap of the way of no return. Avoid it at all costs. Compassion is good; self-pity is a deadly trap.

4. *Fear of the future*: the paralytic man in the story had suffered for a long time. His reality was now so different from his before getting sick. In his mind, questions would come that brought fear, uncertainty, and a lack of hope. His future was not secure; all he knew was he was sick and waiting for someone else to get him to those healing waters. But maybe deep down, he was also afraid of what could happen if he would get healed. If he were to get well, things would have to change. Now, he would have to get a job, the education he never had, or a wife and a family. He would have to change from being a dependent man to a responsible one, providing for himself and his family. That sounds very scary to me. We are all creatures of habit; we like to do what we do now. Change is always scary and uncomfortable. So, if we have been sick for a long time, we have gotten used to being ill. We can control our circumstances because of our sickness. Getting healthy means we must change. If we get well, we will no longer depend on others.

We might have to learn how to drive or walk again. This might mean that we will now contribute financially to the household. We can help our children with our grandchildren because we no longer have arthritis pain that limits our activities. It might mean going back to the workforce or finishing our degree. The sky is the limit regarding the possible results of our healing. But the question remains: do you want to get well? If the answer is yes, we must consider that there might be some fear of what would happen if we got well. We cannot conquer what we cannot confront, and we cannot confront what we cannot see. So, seeing fear of the future is the first step in conquering it. Let us be honest enough to recognize that this might hinder our healing. It is an emotionally invisible barrier that can be demolished if we recognize it as a possibility, accept it, and then stand against it.

So, let us consider whether we have any of these characteristics of the paralytic man in the story.

If we do, let us ask ourselves the question Jesus asked: Do you want to get well? What would happen next can be the miracle that Jesus performed in the story. He commanded the man to get up, pick up his mat and walk. The instructions for our healing may or may be more complex than those. But if we listen carefully, we might get the answers we seek. Restoration of health is possible, and healing can come in many different forms.

CHAPTER 9

Restoring What Was Lost!

Sickness in our bodies has a purpose. When it comes in the form of a chronic disease, it can turn into the most vicious enemy we can ever confront. I see it as a villain whose purpose is to steal, kill, and destroy. Unless we see chronic illness as something that is stealing from us and our families, we will not have enough courage to confront it, battle it, and defeat it.

We must see with a clear vision and recount our losses. This is not so we can wail and waddle in despair or hopelessness, but it is intended to give us a reality check on where we stand.

Chronic illness has a profound effect not only on the lives of those who carry the disease but also on the lives of those around them. Whether family members, spouses, children, friends, or coworkers, they all become affected by the burden of the disease. A medical term and diagnosis is now assigned its own ICD code for medical billing: Caregiver Burden or Caregiver Stress.

Now, it is not only the person suffering from the disease but also those around him who need medical attention.

The burden takes many forms, including financial losses, loss of relationships, loss of independence, and loss of self-esteem.

In this chapter, we will talk about restoring what was lost, but we must start by identifying what we lost first.

It is of extreme importance as well that we go through a mourning process for our losses.

In 1969, Psychiatrist Elizabeth Kubler-Ross identified the five stages of grief: denial, anger, bargaining, depression, and acceptance. She used it with dying patients, their caregivers, and their families. She stated that the stages didn't have to be in a particular order and that some may not go through all of them.

This model doesn't have to be specific for death, but for any loss we experience. We must be aware of what we are going through as we have suffered losses in our journey towards healing.

Recognizing and accepting what we are going through doesn't

mean we won't fight against it, but it does mean we will have an emotionally balanced mindset to be strong enough to continue to fight. Unless we can recognize and express our inner struggles, we won't be able to move forward and keep fighting until we win and recover some losses.

In his book *The Myth of Normal*, Dr. Gabor Matte explains how authenticity can heal trauma and deep emotional wounds and bring physical healing as a result—being authentic starts by asking ourselves questions and realizing where we stand.

Analyzing our emotions, thoughts, and actions will reveal our souls and what damages have occurred. These damages might be evident on the outside but still concealed in our deepest parts.

This journey can be difficult, and it will require support. Do not hesitate to cry out to others; as much as a chronic illness can be very isolating, we must break out from that place into a place of community and love.

If we look around carefully, we will see that we are not alone but surrounded by people who can and will help.

We will explore more of this in the coming chapters.

We must analyze our current losses, mourn over them as long as needed, and then make an action plan to return what belongs to us.

Dottie Osteen, in her book *Healed of Cancer*, describes how, in her healing journey, she would keep looking at images of herself when she was healthy. She would have them all over her house. She would look at herself doing what she enjoyed and look young, vibrant, and slim. With those images, she purposed to regain all that and become healthy again. And it happened!

In her case, she refused all medical intervention and believed a supernatural cure to come her way. I am not suggesting you do the same thing, but what I want you to consider is that having an image of what we want to become will not only sustain us when feeling down, depressed, or anxious but will give us the courage to keep going against the strong current of the disease.

So, let us consider what we lost and what we want to recover.

If sickness has stolen your youth, then propose yourself to regain some of it. Do something small that will take you there. If your finances have been lost, mourn, but get up and see how to recover. Plan to get there. Get professional advice if needed but do something about it. And so on.

Plan on how to recover every area of your life from which you feel the sickness has been stolen. Don't let this sickness get away with anything but fight back. We feel defeated when we look at our bodies, minds, and emotions. We see them as messes we now must deal with, but if we decide not to stay there but move forward, we will.

Starting small is okay; pick one thing and make a small change. Small changes go a long way, but they begin with a decision. Will you make one today? Will you be courageous enough to say yes, I will? Will you restore what was lost?

CHAPTER 10

Healing Is a Journey You Don't Take Alone!

We must identify who's coming with us as we progress through the healing process.

In the previous chapter, we discussed losses and how to restore some of them. Here, we will specifically discuss people who are with or are not with us on this journey.

Some of our losses will be relationships. Maybe you were employed full-time before you got sick and had many relationships daily. You were used to handling multiple tasks and perhaps even had people you supervised. Now, in the middle of your disease, those relationships have dissipated or disappeared; you no longer have a job, no longer have people you supervise, and the world around you has shrunk. You will feel that loss, and it is essential to acknowledge and mourn over it. But once you do that, it is time to see the people who still hang around.

At the beginning of my journey, I had more than enough people who wanted to be near me. People always wanted to visit, pray for me, bring me food, take me to the doctor, and help my family as caregivers. Honestly, it was a bit overwhelming. Being a people-pleaser didn't help. I still wanted to make everyone happy so that I would accept all visitors or help. I am very grateful for all the people who showed me their love. But as the days went by, I felt that my little energy was going into keeping all those people happy and allowing them to come into my life when I had nothing for them. I was still looking into how or what I could give them. I was empty and still wanted to give.

Then something unique happened. I started to say no to visitors, phone calls, and text messages. I began to use the little energy I had to take care of my basic needs. If I needed sleep, I would sleep; if I needed food, I would eat; if I needed prayer, I would pray. And if I needed someone by my side, I would ask for that person. I discovered that only some were beneficial to be by my side. Some would ask many questions I couldn't answer; some would give me answers to questions I didn't ask. But then some would be on standby. Those people became my companions. I learned that a big circle of people is not always the best for those who are sick. My circle became smaller but more effective and loving. Not that the other people were not loving or loving me, but it was impossible to continue connecting to all of them when no part of me was left to connect.

I'm saying here that our healing journey is one we take with others, but we must be selective about who will be privileged to join us.

So, what do I look for in someone who will be by my side on this journey?

1. Honesty

The first quality that a person who comes alongside us must have is honesty. Someone who will not tell us the truth will only hinder us. Now, honesty does not mean rudeness. Some might want to help tell the truth, but they will do it unlovingly.

There are ways of speaking truth in love. The goal is to apply the golden rule. Don't do it to others if you would not say it like that to yourself.

Now, if you have a person in your healing journey, allow those who have truths to say to you, no matter how uncomfortable those might be. They can see a part of you that you cannot see. It is like looking at ourselves in a mirror only from the front. When we have those mirrors where we can see the sides and back, we realize that that dress or suit is not flattering on us.

In my journey, I have the privilege to have honest people around me. In the beginning, when they would tell me something different than what I was thinking, I would not receive it and would get upset at them. Thankfully, they understood my situation and did not get offended by me. They just kept loving me and kept speaking the truth. I finally realized that If I listened to them, I would benefit from their counsel and make progress in my healing.

So, if you have a person or persons in your life who are brave enough to tell you the truth, listen to them. Do not despise their counsel; at least consider it and put your guard down. Just because someone else is not going through what you are going through doesn't mean they don't understand. It is always good to have someone else's perception or viewpoint.

2. Perseverance

I cannot begin to tell you how important perseverance is in someone who will come alongside you while you're sick. The journey might not be as short as we all want, and having someone who will stick around no matter what is very important.

When I first got sick with Myasthenia Gravis, the person closest to me was my husband. Yes, my adult children, sisters, and some very close friends cared for me, but my husband was the closest one. I know he wasn't the most suitable person to understand how to care for or even be patient with me. But one thing he showed was perseverance. No matter how he felt, how tired, and what things he had to give up, he was there for me.

Having a chronic illness is a family thing. Everyone's life changes because of one person being sick, and everyone reacts differently to the situation. But those people who hang out with you, who give up their time, their activities, and their resources to be by you, are precious to the sick person.

So, look around you. Who is always there for you? Who comes back to you even after you have thrown a temper tantrum? Who doesn't mind giving up their time to spend an hour or so by your side, even if you're in a bad mood or severe pain that day? Those people are meant to help you in your healing journey.

3. *Affection*

There is a Bible verse that talks about love. It's even called the love chapter. It describes what love is and what love isn't, but it also says that you can have and be all these other amazing things, but if you have no love, you're nothing. That principle can be applied to the people traveling alongside you. They might be the most qualified caregivers, talented cooks, or entertaining companions, but lacking love and affection will produce little on your healing.

This is particularly important for the chronically ill person who has lost many relationships, resources, and finances due to the illness. Nothing can compensate better for those losses than love. An affectionate relationship will do miracles in the healing process. It can even teach us how to love ourselves better.

For some of us, love has been conditional. By this, I mean we believe that we deserve love because of what we do. But when you are in a state of disease and your body, mind, and emotions cannot give anything to others, receiving unconditional love can make a big difference.

Suddenly, we can see that it doesn't matter what we do, that love has nothing to do with how we behave or what we do or say. That unconditional experience will motivate us to start loving ourselves in the state that we are.

In my case, I didn't like the way the disease was transforming me; I could no longer move the same, speak the same, and even eat the same.

I became a different person because of the things I couldn't do anymore. I started to hate myself and blame myself for changing so much. I liked and loved the person who would do many things all the time, the one who could go for walks, dance, talk, speak at conferences, take care of sick people, etc. But this person was not there anymore.

All I had was someone confined to a bed or wheelchair, someone who needed others for her basic needs. I couldn't cook for myself, couldn't bathe myself, or go anywhere without someone else assisting me. Even conversing with someone, I could only speak for a few minutes before getting exhausted and having no more voice. Eating had also to be limited as I would get highly fatigued and choked at times. But as I saw other people loving on me, not depending on what I would do for them but unconditionally, I began to do the same.

I accepted that I was limited but recognized that I was still the same person, except without all the activities that defined me. Loving myself became my goal. Not blaming myself for being sick was the starting point, but it progressed to forgiveness, acceptance, and a loving relationship with myself.

Ultimately, loving myself transferred into genuinely loving others without asking them to perform to be loved.

4. Courage

Being sick is not for the faint of heart. Sickness threatens to take over your life by stealing peace and creating fear and anxiety. Having someone courageous by your side is a must.

The sick person will be afraid of the current situation and the future, especially if the chronic disease is incurable. So, to travel this journey, we must have a companion who can help us see things differently.

Fear and anxiety are enemies to be defeated in this journey. Bravery, courage, and optimism are the keys to beating them. Seeing the glass half full will help us get up and go.

Courage can be contagious. Courage can be imitated. Courage can be multiplied.

If someone can show a courageous attitude around us, our levels of anxiety will be challenged, and we will have the option to choose to be brave despite our circumstances.

I always enjoy hearing stories of unlikely heroes. Some of these heroes never thought of themselves as such until they decided to do something that required courage. Courage doesn't mean we don't experience fear but move on to do something even if we are afraid.

So, look for someone who does courageous things even when afraid—who will inspire you with her courage despite the circumstances. You will soon discover that instead of fear and anxiety, you will have the courage to continue your journey.

5. *Flexibility*

There might be more qualifications for the people needed for our journey. However, an essential aspect is that the person should be flexible. By this, I mean not only in schedules but in attitudes.

When you have a chronic disease, you are different every day, sometimes every hour or every minute: your mood changes, your levels of physical activity change, your level of engagement changes. As you change so much, your company of people must also be willing to change.

Adapting to you and being flexible to others is essential. You may have planned a doctor's visit that you must reschedule now or a fun outing that you're too sick to attend. The people around you should be sensitive enough to understand and reschedule their plans.

I am very grateful that people around me didn't mind having to move their schedules when mine had to be moved. I still don't drive, so I need people to drive me. That is very humbling for me, as I was always so independent. I have never been a good planner and have difficulty with time management, so the people who help me know by now that when I say 10:00 a.m., it might be 10:10 or even 10:30. So they allow that extra time when they plan to get me.

I am also learning how to be flexible with myself. I never knew with this disease when I was not going to be as strong as I thought, so now, if I am not the strongest, I can say no to the plans I already had.

So, flexibility is an art that we must practice. It will never look the same, but it will give us many opportunities to be different and to adapt to others and others to us. It will create a stronger bond between our relationships that will guarantee us the success we all want as we continue to travel toward our healing.

CHAPTER 11

Wrapping It Up: *Your Commitment*

So far, we have been traveling together as we read about healing chronic illnesses.

In the last chapter, I emphasized that healing is a journey we don't take alone. Many people are involved in healing, and we should all clearly understand the need to create and maintain a good support team.

But in this chapter, we must face it all alone. Regarding healing, only one person can decide whether this journey starts, continues, or ends.

The power of decision-making is one of the most precious things one can have. I remember having my patients and giving them my expert opinion about their conditions. One thing I always made sure I did was ask them if they agreed with my plan of treatment. There is nothing worse than feeling, as a patient, that you must agree with your physician because he's the doctor.

To give humans dignity, we must ask every patient what they

desire and wish regarding their condition. Even when patients have a diagnosis of dementia, we must consider what they would have chosen if their minds were as sharp and focused before the disease.

Today marks the end of this book, but it might also be the start of your journey.

As you read this last chapter, I want you to consider what you want. Not what your doctor wants, what your daughter wants, or what your spouse wants. It would be best if you decided for yourself. You must take this journey one day at a time and decide whether to continue it.

I don't believe saying I want to stop my journey is wrong. Only those who walk in your shoes know how much weight you are carrying.

My mother died of leukemia. She struggled with chronic anemia at the end of her life, amongst other chronic conditions that included osteoporosis, which gave her a couple of vertebral fractures and, hence, chronic pain.

She also had hypertension, well-controlled gastritis, colitis, anxiety, and finally, Alzheimer's dementia (early stages). But when her anemia turned into leukemia, and she began cyclic blood transfusions and eventually chemotherapy, her body couldn't take it anymore.

I was not her primary care person, so I wasn't present when her chemotherapies were going on or witnessed the post-effects of them. But my sister was present; she would take her to treatments and transfusions, and then she would convince her to go back to her house to spend some time with her. She wanted to keep her with her as the symptoms of the chemotherapy were very hard for my mother to bear on her own. She had weakness, nausea, abdominal pain, vomiting, fever, chills, etc.

She was in her late 80s when she encountered this disease. She had always been a strong woman, a leader, and a businesswoman with lots of influence and many friends. But at the end of her life, she was broken, weak, and lonely.

However, something vital in her remained until the end: her dignity. She had always joked around about how she wanted her funeral to be. She even said who she wanted and didn't want there. She was a woman who feared nothing, not even death. So when death approached her, she was ready to face it.

I remember her last hospitalization. She was so weak due to the anemia and the effects of her other chronic diseases on her body that she looked like a little girl. She had lost so much weight, and she was not eating barely anything. She slept many hours during the day and night. She had worsening back pain and had to be on pain medications around the clock. Her mind also failed to remember many things. But she could still remember me and my sisters and our children. My oldest son renamed her Bambina Giovanna; she spent hours with him by her bedside.

One day, she seriously talked to my older sister, Elsa. Elsa had lived all her life with my mom; even after she married, she, her husband, and her daughter lived with her. She was also one of her primary caregivers.

In her last hospitalization and after talking to her oncologist, my mom realized that her medications were not winning the battle against leukemia. The doctor said he could keep giving them to her until the end, but it would not restore her health. He noted the cycles of transfusions would get more and more frequent, and the side effects of chemotherapy would continue to get worse as well. All of this is with the idea of prolonging her life at the expense of her quality of life.

When this was explained to my mom, she immediately knew what she wanted. She said, Stop all treatments, and I am ready to die.

As hard as this seemed to my sisters and me, we had to accept it. She had glimpses of reality where her mind was as clear as that of a healthy person. All her legal documentation about her end-of-life decisions was made at one of those moments.

My sisters and I were named by her medical power of attorney, but she decided to become a DNR (do not resuscitate) patient and stop all her cancer treatments. She became what is called a hospice patient. With this new medical status, we took Mom home, and she died peacefully and comfortably, surrounded by all the people she loved a few weeks later.

This is what I call taking responsibility for ourselves until the end. She demonstrated a courage and character that is seldom seen. She, and only she, decided that her journey was to end sooner rather than later. She knew how she wanted to live, and she certainly knew how she wanted to die.

I am not telling you this story to discourage you but to encourage you. You must be the one that has the wheel of your life. There is someone I trust with my life because of my beliefs. I believe there is a God who is merciful and mighty simultaneously, and I can trust my life to Him and my time to die. But I also know that because of this great love, He has given me free will; that is, I get to decide how to handle my health and make decisions about it.

.

In a previous chapter, I recalled praying and hearing God speak to my heart about my medical condition.

I realized that the way to handle chronic conditions was to seek with all my energy and strength every scientific resource available to me and use and pursue all the spiritual elements of my faith in search of healing. And that's the decision I made. I decided that I would combine the best of both worlds! Science and medicine can offer me many avenues for healing. They all have a cost, and I don't mean just financial cost but time, effort, medication side effects, etc.

What did I have to lose to choose to pursue healing through faith? Maybe some criticism from my peers who think just science is enough? I wasn't, and I'm not worried about that. Faith that perseveres through trials is my main concern.

When we don't see anything happening in front of our eyes, no improvement, but many setbacks, faith in spiritual healing will be tested. But I have seen how this approach has given me back hope, endurance, and perseverance and allowed me to discover many more beautiful aspects of faith.

It is your time to decide what you want to do. How do you want to approach your journey of healing?

After reading this book, you will have a few resources to base your decision on. But whatever that might be, I encourage you to stand firm and persevere. It doesn't matter if the whole world doesn't applaud you; more than likely, they won't. But when it comes to carrying the joy and the pain of a chronic illness, only you get to decide how to do it.

Do not wait for the world to agree; do not wait for your family to decide. Do stand on the shoulders of others who have done it before. Do look for those warriors who have been through months and years of suffering. Some have accomplished breakthroughs, and some have not. Some decided their journeys would continue, and others had to stop.

I want to cheer you on. You might be the one traveling this complicated course of a chronic illness, or maybe you are part of the support team, or perhaps you're even the physician treating the disease or diseases.

Whatever the case, be assured that someone else has already been or will surely be there.

Yes, your shoes might be unique, but look around, and you may find that they look very much like the ones of the person next to you.

Keep traveling this journey, or not; you have the first and the last word.

CHAPTER 12

A Guide for Your Journey!

In the previous chapter, you decided how to travel to pursue healing. But you may need a tour guide with you. There is a difference that has been quoted by many, but the one I heard it from was John Maxwell, a world-recognized author and leadership guru. He said, *you can be a traveling agent or a tour guide.* He said this in the context of leading others.

As you travel on your journey, I believe you will need not a travel agent but a tour guide.

A traveling agent will tell you of the places you will go, what to expect, how much money you will spend, what modes of transportation you will need, etc., but he won't go with you and more than likely he's never been to those places. His information comes solely from studying, researching, and discovering what he brings to you through media and other platforms.

A tour guide, however, can show you more as he is right there with you. He has done it before with other people. He has gone places before he takes you places. His experience is not from books or media; his experience is natural, so he is the best person to be right there next to you.

Let me be that tour guide for you. As we conclude this time together, I want to leave you with some very practical steps to utilize as a thermometer, a compass, and a road map. Use them how and when you believe you're getting a little lost. Use them when discouragement settles in, or you feel helpless or hopeless. Use them to cheer you on, push you forward, quiet you down, and listen.

I have used all or most of them. I could be better, and I have failed many times to be consistent in any or all of them. But I have discovered that once I return and use them, I reset myself to start over again.

Here is to you, hero, soldier, wonderful creation! Let's move along!

1. *FAITH:* The number one ingredient or step in your journey is faith. Faith is believing in something that you do not see. As you carry the disease burden, you must believe in your healing. Faith, in this case, is believing you can get well. As you receive a horrible diagnosis that science has no answer for, yet you must rise above it and have faith. Faith in God, faith

in science, faith in your doctor, or faith in your treatments. This will make you or break you. And if you don't have faith, then borrow it from others. Surround yourself with people who will stand with you and for you. When you see only the worst, have people around you who can see the best and who will refuse to believe there is no hope.

2. *LOVE:* Above all, love. Loving others is almost always easy, but loving ourselves gets messy and complicated. As you navigate this journey, you must recognize if there's any part of you that you are not loving, and you must start loving yourself so much that you will do whatever it takes to improve yourself. Recognize what makes you feel loved by others, and then practice doing the same things yourself. Do you need a quiet time? Please do it. Do you need a bubble bath? Please do it. Do you want to stay in bed a little longer? Please do it. Do you want to treat yourself to a movie? Please do it. Whatever the expression of love is, start doing it consciously.

3. *LAUGH:* Laughter is a good medicine. The art of laughing or the science of laughing can be discussed altogether in another book. Suffice it to say that our hearts get energized and full of hope as we laugh. Surround yourself with people who have a sense of humor and know how to laugh. Laugh at the things you do that you find stupid or funny. Refrain from being so strict with yourself when you make a mistake or even when your doctor makes a mistake. Laugh at him and laugh with him. Laugh together. It will make things easier. And believe me, it cost me a lot to laugh. I would get offended when people around me laughed, and I did not appreciate jokes. But as I took myself less seriously, I began to experience a warmth that would come upon my heart, and things did not matter much anymore. The heart is where everything starts; if it is heavy, serious, and upset, it won't get much better. Let us laugh our way out of our sicknesses.

4. **REFLECT:** When our days are long, and we get confused about the long nights, we can get lost. There are times when the symptoms of the disease linger for hours on end. During the day, it is difficult to eat, to go places, to take a shower, and we long for the night, but then the night gets here, and our bodies are so tired and full of pain or other limitations that we cannot rest. The cycle can continue for days, weeks, or months. It is here where we must actively pause our minds and bodies. We need to make time to reflect on all the things happening around us. We cannot get lost in our symptoms, but we must pause, reflect, and meditate on how we feel, how we think, how we can change things around us when we can, and how to accept that we are limited in some aspects but not in all of them. Taking the time to think is precious.

This will deliver us from the trap of self-pity. Self-pity says: you're doomed, it will never change, you have to feel sorry and curl back into bed. But you can think you're way out of this by reflecting, analyzing, and discovering different ways to counterattack the disease.

5. JOURNAL: After reflection, let's put our thoughts into words. Journaling has been proven to be a release for anxiety, depression, and other mental issues. As we unscramble our minds in reflection, the next step is to put those thoughts on paper (computer, phone, etc). Whatever means you use to document it, please do it. This serves at least two critical goals. One is to record your thoughts before you forget them; the other is to go back and read them to remind yourself of your progress and achievements. The greatest reward you will have in journaling will be remembering the times of struggle that took you to your victory. So, let us journal away our sorrows and turn them into dancing!

6. FRIENDSHIPS: What would I have done without friendships? My friends play such an essential role in my healing journey that I must give you this as a part of the tour guide experience. If you don't have friends, then start being friendly yourself. Many times, chronic diseases make us bitter and resentful. We want to get better, and it seems nothing works.

Our attitude changes, and if we had friends before our disease, we soon begin to separate from them. We don't want them to be affected by our constant complaints and symptoms, and we decide we're better off alone. Big mistake! Do not push your friends away! But welcome them with open arms. They will bring joy, comfort, and support when needed. It is time to do the opposite if you're always giving and never receiving. Learn to receive from your friends. Be honest with them and explain why you're not as engaging as before, but say you still need them around. Tell them that maybe you cannot give a lot right now but are willing to be on the receiving end of their love. And whenever you can express your love and gratitude towards them, do it with simple acts that won't require much from you. Love heals. Let them love you.

7. *FAMILY:* There is nothing like the love of a family. Your family will play a vital role in your healing journey. Take them along with you. Do love them back. Do express your gratitude to them. Do make decisions together and plans together. Your family is also navigating your chronic disease. They also need support and might need to get it outside of you. You cannot carry their burdens; they can only carry yours so much. Give them space to do that. Suggest rotation schedules, involve friends or extended family to go with you to doctor's appointments, treatments, physical therapy, or run

errands. Above all, please get to know them better. This is the time when you will discover amazing things about them. Be amazed at their beauty and their strength. As you reflect on them, please give thanks for them. If you don't have a family, look for one. Alone is not the place to be when you carry the burden of a chronic disease. If you need to reconcile with your family, do so. This is the time to ask and give forgiveness. There's nothing worse than a sick person alone. Look for ways to reconcile, and if not possible, you forgive, move on, and look for a loving family to adopt you. There's always someone willing and capable of loving others in their suffering.

8. *DREAMS*: Dear, to dream again! When the burden of disease becomes unmanageable, it is like a mountain of despair that we cannot possibly move. Our dreams are shattered, broken, displaced, or at best put on hold. It looks impossible to attain the desires of our hearts. When we lose hope, we lose the ability to dream. And by dreaming, I don't necessarily mean natural dreams when we sleep but the dreams of our hearts. Maybe when disease struck you, you were about to start a new business, relationship, or career. Whatever motivated you died when you were diagnosed. But amid tragedy, dreams can take a whole new spin. Go back and look at the things that made you wake up daily. Those things that were about to be birthed became stillborn. It is time to wake up from the slumber of apathy and conformity and challenge yourself to keep dreaming, to dream again, to resurrect the dead dream. It takes but a decision. Once you decide that you still matter and that what you do is important not just for you but for others, you will have the energy to recreate that dream. The dream might look a little different than before; you might need to adapt to the reality of your present situation, but it is still there, waiting to be birthed. You're the only one that carries your dream. Do not let it die; wake it up and resurrect it into life. See your dream impacting others; they are waiting for it.

9. *MOVEMENT:* As you navigate your journey, there will be times, many of them, when the last thing on your to-do list is to move. Pain, weakness, stiffness of your joints, depression, anxiety, many, many symptoms constantly speak to us saying: DO NOT MOVE. Being immobile covers two aspects: our minds and our bodies. Our minds can become quiet and passive, and that's a big no-no. We must keep thinking and innovating; we must continue being creative. Whatever that means to you, use your mind, imagination, and creativity. Maybe you used to like coloring books as a child and then bring that back into your life. Your mind will relax as you focus on the pictures in the book and choose the colors to give

it life. Maybe it is baking, following a recipe, writing poetry, playing a musical instrument, or learning a new language. Our minds need movement; the law of inertia is fundamental when we carry diseases. While we heal, we must keep moving our minds. Our bodies also need movement. Our bodies become slow, stiff, and uncooperative when carrying and navigating this journey. We yearn for the years when we could walk, bike, dance, etc. Those years seem lost, but we must see our bodies and assess their functionality. We do this with the help of healthcare professionals. As we realize our limitations, we will have a starting point for how to become mobile again. Whatever type of movement you can do, do it. If this means moving your toes only, then do it. It means rolling your shoulders, so do it. Start where you're at and move forward. Use mobility devices to enhance your movement. To do things more easily while you work on restoring your mobility. However, this might look like embracing it, so do not be condemned or discouraged because you need a little help. You will see that as you keep moving, your body will respond and cooperate while healing.

10. *PASSION:* I could keep going with this guide, but I will conclude with this last point to get you started. Having a passion for life will keep you steadfast in this challenging journey. Hang on to it; do not let it depart from you. It sounds

easy, but it is easier said than done. This disease that has come to steal from you will also want to steal your passion for life. But a passion is an intense desire that can be maintained amid the most horrible circumstances. Find it, hold on to it. What is your love now? Do you have any left? It all starts with the truth. We cannot change what we cannot accept, and we cannot accept what we cannot see. So, dig into your soul and ask yourself: Where am I? Do I lack passion? Where do I find it? How can I become passionate about life again? It might mean you have to reach out to others; people who lack passion cannot be around others who lack passion. We must rise like eagles if we want to be eagles. We cannot stay on the ground like the chickens pecking away at the dirt, trying to find some worms to satisfy us temporarily but never looking up. Eagles soar; eagles have excellent vision, authority, and majesty. Look around you and see who are the people that you would want to look like. I know you and I are unique originals, but when we go through chronic diseases, we lose even our identity. So, start looking around and see, then keep company with them. Befriend them, reach out, seek advice, study them. Their passion and enthusiasm will rub off on you. Do whatever it takes to renew your love. This will be the fuel that keeps you going; despite all odds, you have hope and a future if you remain passionate about life.

THE END OR NOT...

GENERAL INFORMATION

For information regarding more copies of this book, group orders of this book, lectures, seminars, or presentations with Dr, Diana Carubba, feel free to send an email:

doctorcarubba@gmail.com